LONGEVITY DECODED:

PRECISION LONGEVITY FOR THE REAL WORLD

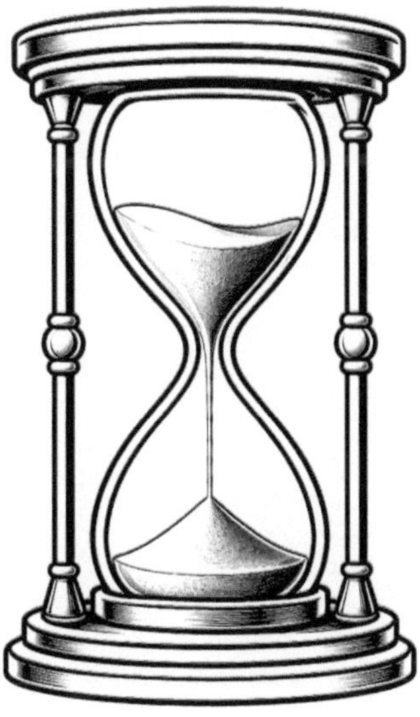

LONGEVITY DECODED:

PRECISION LONGEVITY FOR THE REAL WORLD

We never have enough time with the ones we love.

This book changes that.

Unlock the Life You Were Meant to Live Longer.

DR. PETER BHIRO, DO

PREMIUM EDITION

Published by Immunity Recovery and Regenerative Medicine Center, LLC

First Premium Edition, June 2026

Hardcover ISBN: 979-8-9963520-0-5
Paperback ISBN: 979-8-9963520-1-2

Library of Congress Control Number: LCCN 2026913917

Disclaimer: See full disclaimer page for important medical and legal notices

Contents

Disclaimer

This book is for informational and educational purposes only and is not intended as a substitute for professional medical advice, diagnosis, or treatment. **We do not recommend self-medicating or self-treatment with any substance, supplement, medication, peptide, hormone, or protocol discussed in this book.**

Always seek the guidance of your physician or other qualified health provider with any questions you may have regarding a medical condition or before making any changes to your diet, exercise, supplement, hormone, or medication regimen. The protocols, strategies, and recommendations in this book are based on the author's 29 years of clinical experience and the best available research as of 2026. Individual results vary. What works for one person may not work for another due to genetics, medical history, medications, and lifestyle factors.

Specific Medications and Off-Label Use

References to medications such as rapamycin, peptides (e.g., BPC-157, tesamorelin), low-dose lithium, or other off-label therapies are for informational purposes only. These are powerful tools that require careful medical supervision, regular lab monitoring, and individualized dosing. Unmonitored or high-dose use can lead to serious risks, including immune suppression, hormonal imbalance, cardiovascular complications, and other adverse effects. The author does not endorse self-prescribing or using these without qualified clinical oversight. The author and publisher disclaim any liability for any loss or damage arising from the use of information in this book. Readers assume full responsibility for their health decisions.

Epigraph

We never have enough time with the ones we love.
This book is here to change that.

— Dr. Peter Bhiro

Dedication

To my beloved parents,

who came from a third world country with nothing but dreams and determination.

Your tireless work, endless sacrifices, and unwavering belief in education made my college and medical school possible.

Through your lives you showed me that it is not wealth or material gain that defines a person, but character — integrity, compassion, and kindness toward all — that truly matters.

You taught me that hard work and perseverance can overcome any obstacle.

This book is a testament to the foundation you built.

To my dear brother,

the memory of you and our happy times together continues to inspire me every day.

To my wonderful sister and nephew,

thank you for your constant love and presence in my life.

To my incredible and adorable wife —

your unwavering support, patience, and love have been my anchor through this journey.

You make every step meaningful.

And to my most precious and beautiful daughter — truly a gem and a major inspiration for completing this work.

Your wonderful mind, intelligence, resilience, and spirituality gave me the continued drive I needed to complete this work and bring it to the world.

Above all,

to The Most High, the God of Abraham, Isaac, and Jacob,

and to His Son, my Savior, Yeshua —

You are my strength, my joy, my peace, and the source of all wisdom and purpose.

This book is offered in gratitude for Your guidance and grace.

With all my love and gratitude,

Dr. Peter Bhiro, DO

Preface / Note from the Author

I began this journey in 2013.

I had already spent nearly two decades as a clinician, seeing thousands of patients, witnessing the quiet toll of aging in many of my patients — fatigue, memory fog, loss of strength, the slow erosion of vitality. I started writing pages on longevity, hoping to capture what I saw working in real lives. But life pulled me away — distractions, demands, the daily grind — and the manuscript gathered dust.

Then came 2020 and beyond.

I watched something shift.

Patients returned with new fears: brain fog that wouldn't lift, hearts racing with unexplained arrhythmias, energy that vanished overnight. The surge in cardiovascular and cognitive issues wasn't just statistics — it was real people losing confidence in the usual answers. Traditional medicine offered management, but too often fell short of restoration. People were losing faith, and I felt the weight of that loss.

In that season of challenge, something awakened in me.

The Most High reminded me of the dream He planted years earlier. The pages I started in 2013 weren't lost — they were waiting. With renewed fire, I returned to the work — this time with clarity, urgency, and a deeper mission: to give people hope when it felt too late, and tools that actually worked in the real world.

For 29 plus years I've treated patients — not theories, not lab mice, but human beings. I've seen what sticks, what transforms, what restores. I've watched people in their 80s reclaim vitality, couples regain decades together, families find more time with the ones they love.

That is why this book exists.

Longevity is not about chasing immortality or extreme optimization.

It is about more life — more energy to play with grandchildren, more sharpness to remember shared stories, more strength to walk hand-in-hand with the person you promised forever to.

We never have enough time with the ones we love.

This book is here to change that.

It is written for you — whether you're just beginning, feeling overwhelmed, believing it's "too late," or already on the path and seeking the next edge.

Small, consistent steps compound into extraordinary results.

Hope is not wishful thinking — it is the starting point for real change.

I am grateful to share this with you.

May it bring you the clarity, strength, and years you deserve — and the time to live them fully.

With gratitude and hope,

Dr. Peter Bhiro, DO

January 2026

Acknowledgments

This book would not exist without the many souls who shaped my path.

To my former professor at the A4M, Dr. Pam Smith — a sweet soul whose kindness and encouragement in my early days of Integrative Medicine lit a spark that has never dimmed.

To my undergraduate professor at St. John's University, Dr. William Beckert — whom I cherish deeply. You always pushed me toward excellence and shaped my journey toward medical school. Your belief in me made a lasting difference. May you rest in peace.

To my residency professor at Maimonides Medical Center, Dr. Malcolm Rose — a joy to work with, generous with his extensive knowledge and always welcoming. Your guidance during those formative years meant more than I can express. May you rest in peace.

To my beloved family — my parents, who sacrificed everything to give me education and opportunity; my dear brother, whose memory inspires me daily; my sister and nephew, whose love and presence have been constant; and my incredible wife and beautiful daughter, who have anchored me with unwavering support, patience, and joy through this entire journey. You are both such an inspiration to me, more than you can ever know.

To my patients over the past 29 years — thank you for trusting me with your lives, for teaching me what truly works, and for reminding me every day why hope matters.

And above all, to The Most High, the God of Abraham, Isaac, and Jacob, and to His Son, my Savior, Yeshua — thank You for the vision, the strength, the grace, and the favor that carried this book to completion.

With deepest gratitude,

Dr. Peter Bhiro, DO

Who This Book Is For

This book is for anyone who wants to live stronger, healthier, and longer — no matter where you are starting.

If you're just beginning and feel overwhelmed...

If you think it's "too late" because of age or past choices...

If you're already optimizing and seeking the next evidence-based edge...

Or if you simply want practical tools to feel more alive today —

This book meets you right here.

Longevity is not reserved for the young, the elite, or the perfect. Small, consistent steps, taken from any starting point, compound into extraordinary results.

My goal is simple: to give you hope, clarity, and a realistic path forward. So you can spend more precious time with the people you love.

We never have enough time with the ones we love.

This book is here to change that.

CHAPTER 1

Introduction to Precision Longevity

Aging is not a disease we must accept.

It is a process we can understand, influence, and — to a profound degree — engineer. For too long, we've been told that decline is inevitable: energy fades, memory slips, strength wanes, and the body simply wears out. Conventional or Traditional medicine (Medicine 2.0) excels at treating acute illness, but it often stops at managing chronic conditions rather than preventing or reversing their root causes.

This book is different. It is not about chasing immortality or extreme biohacking.

It is about practical, evidence-based longevity — small, sustainable steps that compound into decades more vitality, clarity, and time with the ones we love. We never have enough time with the ones we love.

This book is here to change that.

The Shift from Medicine 2.0 to Precision Longevity

Conventional medicine (Medicine 2.0) is reactive — it waits for disease to appear, then treats symptoms.

Precision longevity (Medicine 3.0) is proactive — it focuses on **healthspan** (years lived in good health) as much as lifespan.

The goal is simple:

Extend the years we feel strong, sharp, and engaged.

Delay or prevent the diseases of aging (heart disease, cognitive decline, metabolic dysfunction).

Give people more time to live with purpose, love, and connection.

Why Now?

The past few years have exposed cracks in the old model.

Since 2020, clinicians have observed a surge in cardiovascular and cognitive issues — even among those who had **mild or asymptomatic COVID-19** (caused by the SARS-CoV-2 virus). Inflammation, endothelial damage, mitochondrial dysfunction, and accelerated biological aging are no longer theoretical — they are real, measurable, and affecting millions.

Traditional approaches manage these conditions after they appear.

This book aims higher: to **prevent, slow,** and in many cases **reverse** the underlying processes before they become irreversible.

The Pillars of Precision Longevity

This book is built on seven core pillars, each with practical, tiered protocols (Beginner, Intermediate, Advanced):

1. **Sleep, Light, and Circadian Mastery** — The foundation of repair and hormonal balance.
2. **Nutrition** — Evidence over ideology: food as fuel, not dogma.
3. **Exercise** — Sustainable movement that builds resilience without burnout.

4. **Hormonal Mastery** — Optimizing the conductors of energy, repair, and mood.
5. **Cellular Maintenance** — Autophagy, senescence clearance, mTOR balance.
6. **Mitochondrial Resilience** — Powering the cell for decades.
7. **Cognitive & Cardiac Protection** — Safeguarding the brain and heart against modern stressors.

Each chapter offers: (graded honestly — meaning fully transparent about how strong the proof is).

The latest 2026 evidence

Practical protocols for real life.

Hope for every starting point — "it's never too late."

The Promise: You will not find hype, unrealistic protocols, or unproven promises here.

You will find tools that have worked in thousands of real lives — including my own patients over nearly three decades. This is not about living forever.

It is about living well — with energy, clarity, strength, and time for the people and purpose that matter most.

The journey starts now.

With hope and gratitude,

Dr. Peter Bhiro, DO

CHAPTER 2:

Measuring Biological Age: What Actually Works in 2026

If you don't measure it, you can't manage it.

That principle—borrowed from business but perfectly applicable to longevity—is the reason this chapter exists.

Chronological age is the number on your driver's license. Biological age is how old your body actually is at the cellular, tissue, and system level. It's the metric that predicts how long you'll live and how well you'll live.

In 2026, measuring biological age is no longer science fiction or confined to elite research labs. It's accessible, increasingly accurate, and—most importantly—actionable.

But not all tests are created equal.

The market is flooded with options, each claiming to reveal your "true age." Some are grounded in robust science; others are little more than gimmicks. This chapter cuts through the noise to give you the clinician's view: what actually works today, what the latest data says, and how to use these tools to guide your precision longevity protocol.

Chronological vs. Biological Age: The Fundamental Distinction

Chronological age is simple: the number of years since your birth. It's fixed and irreversible.

Biological age is dynamic. It reflects the accumulated damage, repair capacity, and functional reserve of your cells and systems. It can be younger or older than your chronological age—and, crucially, it can be influenced.

Why does this matter?

Because biological age is a far better predictor of remaining healthspan and lifespan than chronological age alone. Studies consistently show that accelerated biological age (when your body is "older" than your calendar years) is associated with higher risks of:

- Cardiovascular disease
- Cancer
- Neurodegenerative disorders
- Frailty
- All-cause mortality

Conversely, a younger biological age correlates with resilience, vitality, and extended high-quality years.

The goal of precision longevity is to slow (and where possible, reverse) the rate of biological aging. But to do that, you need an accurate feedback loop.

The Evolution of Biological Age Clocks

The first practical biological age clocks emerged about a decade ago. Steve Horvath's 2013 epigenetic clock, based on DNA methylation patterns at 353 CpG sites, was groundbreaking. It predicted chronological age with remarkable accuracy and showed deviations in disease states.

Since then, the field has exploded. Second- and third-generation clocks have improved on accuracy, predictive power, and sensitivity to interventions.

Today's leading clocks fall into three main categories:

1. **Epigenetic clocks** (DNA methylation)
2. **Proteomic / multi-omic clocks** (blood proteins, metabolites)
3. **Glycan-based clocks** (inflammation and immune aging)

Each has strengths and limitations. No single clock is "best" for everyone—it depends on your goals.

The Top Clocks in 2026: Head-to-Head Comparison

Here are the leading commercial and research-grade clocks available in 2026, ranked by scientific rigor and practical utility.

Table 2.1: Biological Age Clocks — Key Metrics (2026 Data)

- **GrimAge 2**
  - What it measures: DNA methylation (epigenetic changes)
  - Best for: All-cause mortality prediction
  - Accuracy / Reliability: Very High
  - Cost & Accessibility: Moderate (~$300–$500)
  - Notes: Most predictive of lifespan; updated 2025 version
- **DunedinPACE**
  - What it measures: Pace of aging (rate of biological aging)
  - Best for: Speed of aging over time
  - Accuracy / Reliability: High
  - Cost & Accessibility: Moderate (~$300–$400)
  - Notes: Tracks how fast you're aging (1.0 = normal)
- **PhenoAge**
  - What it measures: Phenotypic age (blood biomarkers + age)
  - Best for: Overall healthspan
  - Accuracy / Reliability: High
  - Cost & Accessibility: Low–Moderate (~$150–$300)
  - Notes: Good for tracking progress
- **Horvath Clock**
  - What it measures: DNA methylation (original pan-tissue clock)
  - Best for: Broad biological age
  - Accuracy / Reliability: Moderate–High
  - Cost & Accessibility: Low (~$100–$250)
  - Notes: Classic, but less specific than newer versions
- **Hannum Clock**
  - What it measures: DNA methylation (blood-based)

- Best for: Blood-based aging
- Accuracy / Reliability: Moderate
- Cost & Accessibility: Low (~$100–$200)
- Notes: Older, but still widely used

- **TruAge (TruDiagnostic)**
  - What it measures: DNA methylation + immune cell composition
  - Best for: Immune aging + biological age
  - Accuracy / Reliability: High
  - Cost & Accessibility: Moderate (~$400–$600)
  - Notes: Consumer-friendly kit; detailed reports
- **Elysium Index**
  - What it measures: DNA methylation (proprietary)
  - Best for: General biological age
  - Accuracy / Reliability: Moderate–High
  - Cost & Accessibility: Moderate (~$500)
  - Notes: Direct-to-consumer, user-friendly
- **GlycanAge**
  - What it measures: IgG glycosylation patterns
  - Best for: Inflammation & immune aging
  - Accuracy / Reliability: Moderate
  - Cost & Accessibility: Moderate (~$350–$500)
  - Notes: Focuses on chronic inflammation
- **Telomere Length**
  - What it measures: Telomere shortening
  - Best for: Cellular aging proxy
  - Accuracy / Reliability: Moderate
  - Cost & Accessibility: Low–Moderate (~$100–$300)
  - Notes: Less predictive alone; better combined
- **NAD+ Levels**
  - What it measures: Cellular energy coenzyme
  - Best for: Mitochondrial & metabolic health
  - Accuracy / Reliability: Moderate
  - Cost & Accessibility: Moderate (~$200–$400)
  - Notes: Emerging, good for tracking interventions

Key Takeaways from the Table:

- **GrimAge v2** remains the gold standard for predicting mortality and disease risk. It's trained on clinical outcomes, not just chronological age.
- **DunedinPACE** is the best for measuring *rate* of aging—ideal for tracking whether your protocol is slowing things down.
- **GlycanAge** excels at capturing inflammation and immune system aging—useful for post-viral or autoimmune patients.
- **TruDiagnostic** offers the most comprehensive report, combining multiple algorithms (including DunedinPACE).

Interpreting Your Results: What the Numbers Mean

A typical report gives:

- Your biological age estimate
- The delta (difference from chronological age)
- Percentile ranking compared to peers
- Specific driver markers (e.g., elevated GrimAge components like PACKYRS for smoking damage or ADM for adrenal stress)

Example interpretation:

- A 48-year-old with a GrimAge of 42 is aging slower than average (good news).
- A 48-year-old with a GrimAge of 55 is aging faster—time to intervene aggressively.

Common patterns I see in clinic:

- High-performers with perfect labs but chronic stress/sleep debt often test 5–10 years older.
- Sedentary individuals with lucky genetics can test younger despite poor habits.
- Interventions (exercise, fasting, sleep optimization) can reverse 3–8 years in 12–18 months—documented in longitudinal studies and my own patient data.

Limitations and Pitfalls

No clock is perfect. Common issues:

- **Test-to-test variability**: The same blood sample sent to different labs can give deltas of 3–5 years. Use the same test for tracking.
- **Snapshot nature**: A single test reflects a moment in time. Stress, infection, or recent travel can skew results.
- **Genetic outliers**: Some people have methylation patterns that make clocks less accurate.
- **Over-reliance**: A number is a tool, not gospel. Integrate with VO2 max, DEXA, bloodwork, grip strength, etc.

How to Use Biological Age Testing in Practice

Recommended protocol:

1. **Baseline**: Choose one primary clock (I favor GrimAge or DunedinPACE for most patients).
2. **Retest**: Every 6–12 months (more frequently if aggressive intervention).
3. **Combine metrics**: Pair with functional tests (VO2 max, muscle mass, fasting insulin).
4. **Prioritize**: If accelerated, double down on foundations (sleep, exercise, nutrition) before exotic therapies.

Closing: The Feedback Loop of Precision Longevity

Measuring biological age is the dashboard for your longevity engine. Without it, you're flying blind.

In 2026, these tools are finally good enough to guide real decisions. Use them wisely, track consistently, and let the data reinforce what works.

> *Next chapter, we tackle the highest-ROI lever of all: sleep and circadian mastery—the foundation everything else is built on.*

CHAPTER 3

The True Foundations: Sleep, Light, and Circadian Mastery

Everything begins with sleep.

If sleep is broken, nothing else matters — hormones crash, inflammation rises, mitochondria weaken, brain fog sets in, and the heart strains.

Sleep is the highest-ROI longevity lever available — free, accessible, and foundational to every other pillar.

This chapter is not about "8 hours or bust."

It is about mastering sleep, light, and circadian rhythm so your body repairs deeply, your energy soars, and your biological age slows.

Why Sleep & Circadian Rhythm Are the True Foundation

During deep sleep, the body:

Clears brain toxins via the glymphatic system (including beta-amyloid linked to cognitive decline).

Releases growth hormone for repair.

Balances cortisol (stress hormone) and melatonin.

Restores autonomic nervous system (HRV improves).

Poor sleep accelerates aging faster than almost any other factor — shortening telomeres, increasing inflammation, impairing insulin sensitivity, and raising risk for heart disease, diabetes, and neurodegeneration.

Light is the master regulator of the circadian clock (suprachiasmatic nucleus in the brain).

Morning bright light sets the rhythm; evening darkness allows melatonin rise.

Modern life inverts this: artificial light at night, dim mornings indoors — resulting in misaligned clocks, poor sleep, and accelerated aging.

Core Principles of Circadian Mastery

1. **Morning Bright Light Exposure**
   - Goal: 10–30 minutes of bright natural light (or 10,000 lux artificial light) within 1 hour of waking.
   - Benefit: Suppresses melatonin, boosts cortisol rhythmically, improves mood/energy, sets strong circadian signal.
2. **Evening Darkness & Blue Light Reduction**
   - Goal: Dim lights after sunset, use blue-blockers (red/orange glasses) 2–3 hours before bed.
   - Benefit: Allows melatonin rise, deeper sleep, better recovery.
3. **Consistent Sleep/Wake Times**
   - Goal: Same bedtime/wake time ±30 minutes, even weekends.
   - Benefit: Stabilizes circadian rhythm, improves HRV and hormonal balance.
4. **Cool, Dark, Quiet Sleep Environment**
   - Goal: Bedroom 60–67°F (15–19°C), pitch black, minimal noise.
   - Benefit: Deeper slow-wave sleep, more growth hormone release.

Practical Protocols (Tiered)

Beginner

- Wake up and get 10 minutes of natural light (open curtains, step outside).

- Dim lights 1 hour before bed, no screens or use blue-blockers.
- Aim for consistent bedtime (even ±1 hour is a win).

Intermediate

- 20–30 minutes morning light exposure (walk outside).
- Strict 2-hour blue light block before bed + red night lights.
- Cool bedroom (use fan/AC) + blackout curtains.

Advanced

- 30+ minutes morning sunlight (or high-lux light panel).
- Full red-light environment after sunset (red bulbs, candles).
- Track sleep/HRV with wearable (Oura/Whoop) — optimize for 20%+ deep sleep.

Common Pitfalls & Fixes

- Late-night scrolling → Fix: Phone in another room after 9 PM.
- Weekend sleep-in → Fix: Wake within 1 hour of weekday time.
- Dim mornings → Fix: Bright light immediately upon waking (even artificial if cloudy).

The Real Impact

Mastering sleep and circadian rhythm alone can improve biological age markers (GrimAge, DunedinPACE) by 2–5 years in 3–6 months — more than most supplements or interventions.

Sleep is not a luxury.

It is the foundation.

Honor it, and every other protocol becomes more powerful.

> *Next chapter: Nutrition for Longevity — evidence over ideology.*

CHAPTER 4:

Nutrition for Longevity — Evidence Over Ideology

Nutrition is the most confusing and divisive pillar of longevity.

Diets are weaponized: keto vs. vegan, carnivore vs. plant-based, intermittent fasting vs. three meals a day. Everyone claims "the truth," yet the evidence tells a simpler story.

This chapter cuts through the noise with one guiding principle:

Evidence over ideology.

We focus on what actually moves the needle for healthspan — not dogma, not trends, not what sells supplements.

Core Principles of Longevity Nutrition

1. **Real Food First**
   Prioritize whole, minimally processed foods — vegetables, fruits, nuts, seeds, quality proteins, healthy fats. Avoid ultra-processed junk (sodas, chips, fast food, packaged snacks).
2. **Time-Restricted Eating (TRE)**
   Limit eating window to 8–12 hours daily (e.g., 10 AM–6 PM).
   Benefit: Improves insulin sensitivity, boosts autophagy, reduces inflammation — even without calorie restriction.

3. **Protein Quality & Timing**
   Aim for 1.2–1.6 g/kg body weight (higher end for active/older adults). Focus on complete proteins (animal sources, soy, quinoa) — distribute across meals for muscle maintenance.
4. **Healthy Fats**
   Emphasize monounsaturated (olive oil, avocados, nuts) and omega-3s (fatty fish, algae oil).
   Limit saturated fats from processed meats; avoid trans fats entirely.
5. **Polyphenols & Fiber**
   Colorful plants (berries, leafy greens, cruciferous veggies) for antioxidants and gut health.
   Fiber (30+ g/day) feeds microbiome, lowers inflammation.
6. **Low Glycemic Load**
   Minimize refined carbs/sugars — keep blood sugar stable to reduce glycation and insulin spikes.

Practical Protocols (Tiered)

Beginner

- Eat real food 80% of the time.
- Try 12-hour TRE (e.g., 8 AM–8 PM eating window).
- Add one extra serving of vegetables daily.
- Swap soda for water or herbal tea.

Intermediate

- 10-hour TRE (e.g., 10 AM–8 PM).
- Protein 1.2–1.6 g/kg, spread over 3 meals.
- Olive oil + fatty fish 3–4x/week.
- 30+ g fiber daily (track with app like Cronometer).

Advanced

- 8-hour TRE (e.g., 12 PM–8 PM).
- Optimize omega-3: 2–4 g EPA/DHA daily.

- Polyphenol-rich foods (berries, dark chocolate, green tea) daily.
- Periodic fasting-mimicking diet (FMD) 2–4x/year (monitored).

Common Pitfalls & Fixes

- **Over-restriction** → Fix: Focus on adding good foods, not banning everything.
- **Weekend binges** → Fix: Keep TRE window consistent (±1 hour).
- **Supplement obsession** → Fix: Food first — supplements only fill gaps (e.g., omega-3 if no fish).

The Real Impact:

Nutrition done right can improve biological age markers (GrimAge, DunedinPACE) by 3–7 years in 6–12 months — more than most drugs or interventions. It reduces inflammation, stabilizes blood sugar, feeds the gut microbiome, and supports every other pillar.

Food is medicine — choose wisely, eat with joy, and let it fuel the life you want to live longer.

> *Next chapter: Exercise as Medicine — sustainable protocols that move the needle.*

CHAPTER 5:

Exercise as Medicine — Sustainable Protocols That Move the Needle

Exercise is not punishment. It is medicine — the most powerful, free, accessible tool to slow aging, reverse decline, and extend healthspan.

This chapter is not about extreme gym sessions or marathon training.

It is about sustainable, evidence-based movement that builds resilience, protects the heart and brain, and fits real life — whether you're 30 or 80, starting from zero or already active.

Why Exercise Is the Ultimate Longevity Lever

- VO_2 Max (maximal oxygen uptake) is the single strongest predictor of all-cause mortality — stronger than smoking, blood pressure, or cholesterol.
- Each 1-MET increase in fitness reduces mortality risk by 12–15%.
- Zone 2 training improves mitochondrial function, endothelial health, insulin sensitivity, and HRV.
- Strength training preserves muscle mass, bone density, and metabolic health — critical after age 40.
- Movement reduces inflammation, boosts BDNF (brain-derived neurotrophic factor), and clears senescent cells.

The data is overwhelming: consistent, moderate exercise outperforms most drugs and supplements for healthspan.

Core Principles of Sustainable Exercise

1. **Zone 2 Cardio** (the foundation)
   - 60–70% max heart rate (conversational pace — can talk but not sing).
   - Benefit: Builds mitochondrial density, improves fat oxidation, protects heart/brain.
2. **Strength Training**
   - Focus on compound movements (squats, deadlifts, presses, pulls).
   - Benefit: Preserves muscle, boosts testosterone/GH, strengthens bones.
3. **Mobility & Stability**
   - Daily stretching, balance work, walking.
   - Benefit: Prevents injury, maintains function into old age.
4. **Consistency Over Intensity**
   - 3–5 sessions/week beats 1–2 extreme ones.
   - Benefit: Sustainable habits = lifelong results.

Practical Protocols (Tiered)

Beginner

- Daily 20–30 min brisk walk (Zone 2 — conversational pace).
- 2x/week bodyweight strength: push-ups (knee if needed), squats, planks (20–30 sec holds).
- Goal: Build habit, feel more energy in 4–6 weeks.

Intermediate

- Zone 2 cardio 3–4x/week (30–60 min walk, cycle, or row).
- Strength 3x/week: dumbbells/bodyweight — 3 sets of 8–12 reps (push, pull, squat, hinge).

- Add 10 min mobility (yoga/stretching) daily.
- Goal: Improved VO_2 max, better labs in 3–6 months.

Advanced

- Zone 2 4–5x/week (45–90 min).
- Strength 3–4x/week: progressive overload (weights increasing).
- Optional HIIT 1x/week (short bursts for mitochondrial boost).
- Track VO_2 max/HRV with wearable.
- Goal: Peak healthspan, biological age reversal.

Common Pitfalls & Fixes

- **Overdoing it** → Fix: Start slow, add 10% weekly max.
- **Skipping recovery** → Fix: Rest days + sleep priority.
- **Boredom** → Fix: Mix activities (walk, swim, bike, dance).

The Real Impact

Consistent exercise can improve biological age markers (GrimAge, DunedinPACE) by 5–10 years in 6–12 months — more than most interventions.

It protects the heart, sharpens the brain, and gives you more years of active, joyful living.

Movement is medicine — take it daily, and live longer with the ones you love.

Next chapter: Hormonal Mastery — optimizing the conductors of energy and repair.

CHAPTER 6:

Hormonal Mastery

Hormones are the conductors of the longevity orchestra.

When balanced, they drive energy, repair, resilience, mood, libido, and metabolic health. When dysregulated, they accelerate aging — muscle loss, fat gain, fatigue, cognitive decline, and disease risk.

This chapter is different.

We focus on evidence-graded, sustainable mastery — lifestyle first, targeted support when needed, legal and safe off-label options for advanced cases. From the 30-year-old with low energy to the 70-year-old seeking vitality — practical paths for all.

The Key Players

1. **Testosterone** (men and women)
   - Drives muscle, bone, libido, mood, metabolic health.
2. **Estrogen/Progesterone** (women primary, men via aromatization)
   - Bone, brain, cardiovascular protection; progesterone aids sleep and neuroprotection.
3. **Thyroid** (T4/T3)
   - Metabolic rate, energy, cognition.
4. **Growth Hormone/IGF-1 Axis**
   - Repair, muscle, recovery.

5. **Cortisol/DHEA**
   - Stress response and resilience.
6. **Insulin**
   - Metabolic switch and anabolic signaling.
7. **Pregnenolone**
   - Neurosteroid precursor; supports cognition, mood, hormone production.

The Evidence: What Actually Moves the Needle

- **Lifestyle levers** (sleep, strength training, Zone 2, nutrition) raise testosterone 15–30% and optimize thyroid/IGF-1 naturally — stronger than most supplements.
- **TRT** (testosterone replacement): Robust data for symptomatic hypogonadism — muscle, mood, libido gains; CVD risk neutral in modern studies.
- **Thyroid optimization**: T3/T4 replacement improves energy, cognition, metabolism when deficient.
- **Peptides** (e.g., tesamorelin, sermorelin, BPC-157): Growing evidence for GH pulse restoration, repair, gut health — legal off-label with monitoring.
- **Cortisol management**: Chronic elevation accelerates aging; sleep/ Zone 2/mindfulness lower it effectively.
- **Pregnenolone/Progesterone**: Supportive for cognitive/mood balance and hormone cascade; evidence emerging but promising in integrative practice.

Practical Protocols: Tiered for Every Starting Point

For those feeling "off" or starting optimization:

- Baseline labs (examples of key markers — not exhaustive; full hormonal work-up may include additional tests): Total/free testosterone, SHBG, estradiol, TSH/free T3/T4/reverse T3/TPO/

TSI antibodies, fasting insulin, morning cortisol, DHEA-S, IGF-1/IGFBP-3, pregnenolone, progesterone.

- Lifestyle first: Sleep 7–9 hours, strength training 3x/week, Zone 2 cardio, protein 1.6 g/kg, healthy fats.

Table 6.1: Hormonal Optimization — Evidence-Graded Interventions

- **Testosterone**
    - Lifestyle Lever (Tier 1): Strength training, sleep, vitamin D, zinc
    - Targeted Support (Tier 2): TRT (gel/injection) if low/symptomatic
    - Advanced (Tier 3): Peptides (e.g., gonadorelin)
    - Evidence Strength: High (lifestyle/TRT)
- **Thyroid**
    - Lifestyle Lever (Tier 1): Iodine, selenium, stress reduction
    - Targeted Support (Tier 2): Levothyroxine or combo T4/T3 if needed
    - Advanced (Tier 3): Desiccated thyroid (off-label)
    - Evidence Strength: High
- **GH/IGF-1**
    - Lifestyle Lever (Tier 1): Intermittent fasting, HIIT, sleep
    - Targeted Support (Tier 2): Secretagogues (tesamorelin, ipamorelin)
    - Advanced (Tier 3): Recombinant GH (rare, monitored)
    - Evidence Strength: Moderate-High
- **Cortisol**
    - Lifestyle Lever (Tier 1): Sleep priority, Zone 2, mindfulness
    - Targeted Support (Tier 2): Phosphatidylserine, ashwagandha
    - Advanced (Tier 3): Low-dose hydrocortisone (adrenal cases)
    - Evidence Strength: Moderate
- **Pregnenolone**
    - Lifestyle Lever (Tier 1): Sleep, stress reduction
    - Targeted Support (Tier 2): Supplementation (10–50 mg)
    - Advanced (Tier 3): Higher dosing with monitoring
    - Evidence Strength: Moderate

- **Progesterone**
  - Lifestyle Lever (Tier 1): Sleep, magnesium
  - Targeted Support (Tier 2): Bioidentical (women, or men if low)
  - Advanced (Tier 3): Advanced balancing protocols
  - Evidence Strength: Moderate

Clinician Caveats

- **Test, don't guess**: Labs before/after interventions.
- **Individualize**: Women need estrogen/progesterone balance; men monitor estradiol.
- **Safety**: Avoid **unmonitored or high-dose protocols** — rogue or poorly supervised practices can lead to serious risks, including erythrocytosis, estrogen imbalance, cardiovascular events, and potential cancer acceleration. Always work with qualified, experienced clinicians who prioritize regular monitoring, evidence-based dosing, and patient safety.
- **Age matters**: Optimization goals shift — vitality in 40s, preservation in 70s.

The Real Impact

Balanced hormones aren't about "feeling 25 again."

They're about **feeling alive** — sharp, strong, resilient — at any age.

Patients who master this report renewed energy and well-being.

Start with lifestyle.

Add targeted support when needed.

Monitor and adjust.

Next chapter: Cellular Maintenance — autophagy, senescence, and the cleanup crew.

CHAPTER 7:

Cellular Maintenance: Autophagy, Senescence, mTOR

The hallmarks of aging don't operate in isolation.

Cellular "housekeeping" — clearing damage, removing dysfunctional components, and regulating growth pathways — is where many interventions converge.

This chapter covers the core systems:

- **Autophagy**: Cellular recycling and cleanup.
- **Senescent cells**: "Zombie" cells that accumulate and inflame.
- **mTOR** (mechanistic target of rapamycin): The growth vs. repair switch.

We grade the evidence, separate promise from proof, and provide practical, sustainable tools — from lifestyle to advanced options.

No extremes. Just what works in the real world.

Autophagy: The Cellular Recycling System

Autophagy ("self-eating") removes damaged proteins and organelles, maintaining cellular health.

- **Evidence**: Strong in animals (lifespan extension); human data shows improved biomarkers (lower inflammation, better insulin sensitivity) with inducers like fasting.
- **Inducers**: Intermittent fasting/TRE (Chapter 4), exercise (Chapter 5), spermidine-rich foods, rapamycin (below).

Senescent Cells: Clearing the Zombies

Senescent cells stop dividing but secrete inflammatory factors (SASP) that drive aging.

- **Evidence**: Senolytics clear them in mice, improving healthspan; small human trials show reduced senescence markers and improved physical function.
- **Senolytics**: Fisetin, quercetin, dasatinib (intermittent); emerging options like navitoclax.

mTOR: The Growth-Repair Balance

mTOR (mechanistic target of rapamycin) drives growth when nutrients are abundant, repair when scarce.

- **Evidence**: Inhibition extends lifespan in animals; human data from rapamycin shows immune benefits and potential healthspan extension (PEARL trial updates 2025–2026).
- **Inhibitors**: Rapamycin (low-dose intermittent), lifestyle (fasting, protein cycling).

Table 7.1: Cellular Maintenance Interventions — Evidence-Graded

- **Intermittent Fasting/TRE**
  - Mechanism: Boosts autophagy
  - Evidence Strength (Human): High
  - Practical Use: Daily or periodic (Chapter 4)
  - Notes: Sustainable, low-cost
- **Spermidine**
  - Mechanism: Autophagy induction
  - Evidence Strength (Human): Moderate

  - Practical Use: Foods (wheat germ) or supplement 1–10 mg
  - Notes: Observational mortality reduction
- **Fisetin/Quercetin**
  - Mechanism: Senolytic (clear zombie cells)
  - Evidence Strength (Human): Promising
  - Practical Use: Intermittent high-dose (e.g., 20 mg/kg fisetin 2 days/month)
  - Notes: Small trials show reduced inflammation
- **Rapamycin**
  - Mechanism: mTOR inhibition
  - Evidence Strength (Human): Moderate-High
  - Practical Use: Low-dose intermittent (off-label, monitored)
  - Notes: Immune benefits; ongoing trials

Practical Application

- **Beginner:** Prioritize sleep, Zone 2 exercise, TRE — strong autophagy without supplements.
- **Intermediate:** Add spermidine-rich foods, periodic FMD.
- **Advanced:** Consider senolytics or low-dose rapamycin with clinician monitoring.

Clinician Caveats

- Test markers: Inflammatory cytokines, biological age clocks pre/post.
- Safety: Senolytics/rapamycin can suppress immunity short-term — not for everyone.
- Individualize: Cancer history, autoimmune conditions require caution.

The Real Impact

Effective cellular maintenance doesn't reverse aging overnight.

It slows accumulation of damage, reducing inflammation and preserving function — the quiet engine behind vitality.

Combine with foundations (sleep, exercise, nutrition) for synergy.

> *Next chapter: Mitochondrial Resilience — powering the cell for decades.*

CHAPTER 8:

Mitochondrial Resilience

Mitochondria are the power plants of your cells — and the Achilles' heel of aging.

They generate 90% of your energy (ATP), regulate metabolism, and control cellular signaling. When they function well, you feel sharp, strong, and resilient. When they falter, fatigue, inflammation, and disease follow.

Mitochondrial dysfunction is a hallmark of aging: fewer mitochondria, more damage, less efficiency.

This chapter is about protecting and restoring them — with sustainable, evidence-based tools.

No extremes. Just what works in the real world.

The Evidence: Why Mitochondria Matter for Longevity

- Energy decline: Mitochondrial capacity drops 10% per decade after 30.
- Disease link: Dysfunction implicated in neurodegeneration, cardiovascular disease, diabetes, cancer.
- Longevity signals: Interventions improving mitochondrial health (e.g., Zone 2 exercise, NAD+ support) correlate with better biomarkers and lower mortality.

- Human data: 2025–2026 trials show improved mitochondrial markers (e.g., PGC-1α expression) with lifestyle and targeted compounds.

The Core Strategies

1. **Lifestyle Levers (Tier 1 — Highest ROI)**
    - Zone 2 exercise (Chapter 5): Stimulates mitochondrial biogenesis via PGC-1α.
    - Intermittent fasting/TRE (Chapter 4): Triggers mitophagy (mitochondrial cleanup).
    - Sleep and circadian alignment (Chapter 3): Essential for mitochondrial repair.
    - Cold/heat exposure: Mild stress (sauna, cold showers) activates resilience pathways.
2. **Nutrients and Compounds (Tier 2)**
    - NAD+ precursors (NMN/NR): Boost NAD+ levels; small human trials show improved mitochondrial function.
    - Urolithin A: Activates mitophagy; trials show better muscle mitochondrial health.
    - PQQ: Promotes new mitochondria; early data promising.
    - CoQ10/Magnesium: Support electron transport chain.
3. **Advanced Options (Tier 3 — Monitored)**
    - Red light therapy: Low-level wavelengths improve mitochondrial efficiency.
    - Mitochondrial peptides (e.g., SS-31): Emerging for repair.

Biological Age Clocks & Mitochondrial Support

- **Zone 2 Exercise**
    - Mechanism: PGC-1α biogenesis
    - Evidence Strength (Human): Very High
    - Practical Use: 3–4 sessions/week (Chapter 5)
    - Notes: Highest ROI, sustainable
- **TRE/Fasting**
    - Mechanism: Mitophagy
    - Evidence Strength (Human): High

- Practical Use: Daily or periodic (Chapter 4)
- Notes: Low-cost, synergistic

- **NMN/NR**
  - Mechanism: NAD+ restoration
  - Evidence Strength (Human): Moderate-High
  - Practical Use: 500–1,000 mg/day
  - Notes: Raises NAD+; metabolic benefits
- **Urolithin A**
  - Mechanism: Mitophagy activation
  - Evidence Strength (Human): Promising
  - Practical Use: 500–1,000 mg/day
  - Notes: Gut microbiome dependent
- **PQQ**
  - Mechanism: New mitochondria
  - Evidence Strength (Human): Moderate
  - Practical Use: 10–20 mg/day
  - Notes: Synergistic with CoQ10
- **Red Light Therapy**
  - Mechanism: Cytochrome c oxidase
  - Evidence Strength (Human): Moderate
  - Practical Use: 10–20 min sessions
  - Notes: Home devices available

Practical Application

- **Beginner**: Prioritize Zone 2 walks, sleep, TRE — massive mitochondrial benefits without supplements.
- **Intermediate**: Add NMN/NR or urolithin A if labs show low energy markers.
- **Advanced**: Layer red light, PQQ, monitored peptides.

Clinician Caveats

- **Test markers**: ATP production proxies (organic acids), NAD+ levels, mitochondrial antibodies if suspected dysfunction.
- **Individualize**: Mitochondrial issues common in chronic fatigue, neurodegeneration.
- **Safety**: High-dose NAD+ precursors can cause flushing; start low.

The Real Impact

Healthy mitochondria don't just give energy — they give **vitality**.

The difference between dragging through the day and thriving through decades.

Protect them with foundations.

Support them when needed.

> *Next chapter: Cognitive Longevity — building a brain that lasts.*

CHAPTER 9:

Cognitive Longevity: Building a Brain That Lasts

Cognitive decline is the fear that looms largest in aging — losing memories, sharpness, independence, the essence of who we are.

Yet the brain is remarkably resilient. With the right strategies, we can protect it, build reserve, and even improve function well into later decades.

This chapter addresses one of the most urgent concerns today: the rise in cognitive issues since COVID, alongside proven and promising ways to safeguard the brain.

We separate proven foundations from emerging non-traditional approaches — lifestyle first, targeted support when needed.

No extremes. Just practical, sustainable paths to a brain that lasts.

The Post-COVID Cognitive Challenge — and the Path Forward

Since 2020, clinicians have observed increased cognitive complaints and dementia risk, even in mild or asymptomatic COVID-19 cases (caused by SARS-CoV-2).

- **Evidence**: Large cohorts show higher risk of new-onset dementia; mechanisms include neuroinflammation, vascular damage, blood-brain barrier disruption, and persistent effects.
- **Real-world impact**: Many patients report "brain fog," memory issues, or accelerated decline — eroding faith in conventional approaches focused on symptom management.

This is where integrative strategies shine — addressing root inflammation, mitochondrial function, and neuroprotection often yields better outcomes than waiting for decline.

The Evidence: What Drives Cognitive Decline and Protection

Alzheimer's disease (AD) accounts for 60–70% of dementia cases, characterized by amyloid-β plaques, tau tangles, neuroinflammation, vascular damage, and neuronal loss.

Key modifiable risks (Lancet Commission 2024–2026 updates):

- Hypertension, diabetes, obesity, inactivity, isolation, hearing loss — addressing these could prevent/delay ~45% of cases.

2025–2026 breakthroughs:

- Multidomain interventions (FINGER, POINTER updates): Lifestyle programs improve cognition even in APOE ε4 carriers — outperforming drugs in prevention.
- Anti-amyloid therapies (lecanemab, donanemab): Slow early AD; prevention trials ongoing.
- Blood biomarkers: Plasma p-tau217/Aβ42 ratio highly accurate for amyloid positivity.

Lifestyle remains the strongest lever.

Core Foundations (Tier 1 — Highest Evidence)

1. **Exercise** (Chapter 5)
   - Zone 2 + strength: Increases BDNF, hippocampal volume, blood flow; reduces amyloid/tau.
2. **Nutrition** (Chapter 4)
   - Mediterranean/MIND diet: 30–50% lower AD risk; omega-3 (DHA), polyphenols, low glycemic.
3. **Sleep** (Chapter 3)
   - Glymphatic clearance removes amyloid; poor sleep accelerates decline.
4. **Cognitive & Social Engagement**
   - Learning new skills, social connections: Build reserve, reduce isolation risk.
5. **Vascular Health**
   - Control blood pressure, cholesterol, diabetes — major drivers of mixed dementia.

Biomarkers & Testing Roadmap

- **When to test**: High risk (family history, post-COVID symptoms, APOE concern) or symptomatic.
- **Key markers** (examples — clinician-guided):
  - Plasma p-tau217/Aβ42 ratio (high accuracy for amyloid).
  - APOE genotyping (risk stratification).
  - Inflammatory markers (hs-CRP, IL-6).
  - Metabolic (fasting insulin, HbA1c).

Use selectively — avoid unnecessary anxiety.

Non-Traditional Strategies (Tier 2–3 — Emerging Evidence)

- **Ketogenic Approaches**
  - Ketones as alternative fuel; trials show cognitive benefit in MCI, especially APOE ε4 non-carriers.
- **Omega-3 (DHA/EPA)**
  - Reduces inflammation; higher intake linked to lower risk, especially with APOE testing.
- **Lion's Mane Mushroom**
  - Promotes NGF; small trials show memory improvement.
- **Red Light Therapy**
  - Improves mitochondrial function, blood flow; early data for mild cognitive impairment.
- **Hyperbaric Oxygen Therapy (HBOT)**
  - Increases oxygenation; trials show cognitive gains in post-stroke/vascular dementia.
- **Sauna & Cold Exposure**
  - Heat shock proteins, improved vascular function; observational links to lower dementia risk.
- **Peptides & Advanced**
  - Cerebrolysin, dihexa (early); monitored only.

Cognitive Protection — Evidence-Graded

- **Multidomain Lifestyle**
  - Mechanism: BDNF, reduced inflammation
  - Evidence Strength: Very High
  - Practical Use: Diet + exercise + social (FINGER/POINTER)
  - Notes: Prevents ~45% cases
- **Omega-3 (DHA)**
  - Mechanism: Membrane health, anti-inflammatory
  - Evidence Strength: High
  - Practical Use: Fatty fish or 1–2g supplement
  - Notes: Stronger in APOE ε4 carriers

- **Ketogenic Diet**
  - Mechanism: Alternative fuel, reduced amyloid
  - Evidence Strength: Moderate-High
  - Practical Use: Low-carb or MCT oil
  - Notes: Benefit in MCI
- **Lion's Mane**
  - Mechanism: NGF promotion
  - Evidence Strength: Moderate
  - Practical Use: 1–3g/day extract
  - **Notes: Small human trials**
- **Red Light Therapy**
  - Mechanism: Mitochondrial boost
  - Evidence Strength: Promising
  - Practical Use: 10–20 min sessions
  - Notes: Home devices
- **Sauna**
  - Mechanism: Heat shock proteins
  - Evidence Strength: Moderate
  - Practical Use: 4–7x/week
  - Notes: Finnish studies lower risk
- **HBOT**
  - Mechanism: Oxygenation, angiogenesis
  - Evidence Strength: Promising
  - Practical Use: Monitored sessions
  - Notes: Emerging for vascular dementia

Practical Application

- Beginner: Sleep, daily walk, Mediterranean eating, social connections — foundation prevents most decline.
- Intermediate: Add omega-3, cognitive training apps, sauna.
- Advanced: Ketones, red light, monitored peptides; plasma testing for personalization.

Clinician Caveats

- Test thoughtfully: Biomarkers for high-risk or symptomatic; avoid unnecessary worry.
- Individualize: APOE ε4 carriers may benefit more from omega-3/ ketones.
- Safety: Non-traditional (HBOT, high-dose supplements) require monitoring.

The Real Impact

A resilient brain isn't about "never forgetting" — it's about staying sharp enough to enjoy life, relationships, purpose.

Start early.

Build reserve.

Protect fiercely.

> *Next chapter: Cardiac Resilience — safeguarding the engine of life.*

CHAPTER 10:

Cardiac Resilience: Protecting Your Heart for Decades

The heart is the engine of life — and one of the most vulnerable targets of aging and modern stressors.

Cardiovascular disease remains the leading cause of death worldwide, and since 2020, clinicians have observed a troubling surge: increased events, inflammation-driven atherosclerosis, autonomic dysfunction, and sudden cardiac issues — even in younger individuals.

This chapter confronts that reality head-on, then pivots to hope.

We focus on resilience — building a heart that withstands stress, recovers strength, and powers vitality for decades.

Lifestyle foundations remain supreme, augmented by targeted non-traditional strategies when needed.

No extremes. Just what works in the real world.

The Post-COVID Cardiac Challenge — and the Path Forward

Since 2020, large cohorts show elevated cardiovascular risk post-COVID-19 (caused by SARS-CoV-2) — higher myocardial injury, arrhythmias, and long-term events, even in mild cases.

Mechanisms:

Endothelial dysfunction and microclots.

Persistent inflammation.

Autonomic imbalance (HRV reduction — heart rate variability, a measure of nervous system resilience).

Accelerated plaque progression.

Traditional cardiology excels at acute intervention, but often has limited tools for deeper reversal, regeneration, or addressing root-cause inflammation and metabolic dysfunction. This is where integrative strategies shine — targeting inflammation, mitochondrial function, and tissue repair frequently yields better functional outcomes and renewed patient hope.

The Evidence: Core Drivers and Protectors

Key modifiable factors:

Inflammation (hs-CRP, IL-6).
Insulin resistance/metabolic syndrome.
Oxidative stress and mitochondrial dysfunction.
Endothelial health (nitric oxide bioavailability).

Protective interventions (2025–2026 updates):

VO_2 max: Strongest predictor of cardiac mortality — each 1-MET gain reduces risk 13–15%.

Zone 2 exercise: Improves endothelial function, HRV, mitochondrial efficiency.

Omega-3, polyphenols: Reduce plaque inflammation.

Sleep and stress mastery: Restore autonomic balance.

Core Foundations (Tier 1 — Highest ROI)

1. **Exercise** (Chapter 5)
   - Zone 2 supremacy: Builds VO_2 max, endothelial health, HRV.
   - Strength for metabolic support.
2. **Nutrition** (Chapter 4)
   - Mediterranean/MIND pattern: Olive oil, fatty fish, berries, nuts — lower CVD mortality 20–30%.
3. **Sleep & Circadian** (Chapter 3)
   - Critical for HRV and inflammation control.
4. **Stress Mastery**
   - Mindfulness, nature, social connection — lowers cortisol-driven damage.

Biomarkers & Testing Roadmap

- **Standard**: Lipids (LDL, HDL, triglycerides), blood pressure, fasting glucose.
- **Advanced** (examples — clinician-guided):
  - Lp(a), ApoB, hs-CRP.
  - NMR lipoprofile (particle size/number — better predictor than standard lipids).
  - Coronary artery calcium (CAC) score.
  - Endothelial markers (FMD if available).
  - HRV monitoring.

Use selectively — guide intervention, track progress.

Non-Traditional Strategies (Tier 2–3 — Emerging Evidence)

- **Omega-3 (EPA/DHA)**
  - High-dose (2–4g): Reduces triglycerides, plaque inflammation.
- **CoQ10**
  - Mitochondrial support; benefits in heart failure trials.
- **Magnesium**
  - Rhythm, blood pressure, endothelial function.
- **Taurine**
  - Anti-arrhythmic, antioxidant; emerging for post-COVID support.
- **Nattokinase**
  - Fibrinolytic; promising for clot/inflammation reduction.
- **Red Light Therapy/Sauna**
  - Improves circulation, NO production.
- **Peptides** (e.g., BPC-157, TB-500)
  - Tissue repair; emerging for cardiac recovery (monitored).

Cardiac Protection — Evidence-Graded

- **Zone 2 Exercise**
  - Mechanism: VO_2 max, endothelial health
  - Evidence Strength: Very High
  - Practical Use: 3–4 sessions/week
  - Notes: Strongest mortality reduction
- **Omega-3 (EPA/DHA)**
  - Mechanism: Anti-inflammatory, triglyceride ↓
  - Evidence Strength: High
  - Practical Use: Fatty fish or 2–4g supplement
  - Notes: Post-COVID inflammation support
- **Mediterranean Diet**
  - Mechanism: Polyphenols, healthy fats
  - Evidence Strength: High
  - Practical Use: Daily emphasis
  - Notes: 20–30% lower CVD risk

- CoQ10
  - Mechanism: Mitochondrial support
  - Evidence Strength: Moderate-High
  - Practical Use: 100–300 mg/day
  - Notes: Heart failure benefit
- Taurine
  - Mechanism: Antioxidant, anti-arrhythmic
  - Evidence Strength: Moderate
  - Practical Use: 1–3g/day
  - Notes: Emerging post-COVID
- Nattokinase
  - Mechanism: Fibrinolytic
  - Evidence Strength: Promising
  - Practical Use: 100–200 mg/day
  - Notes: Clot support
- Sauna
  - Mechanism: Heat shock, circulation
  - Evidence Strength: Moderate
  - Notes: Lower cardiac events in cohorts
- **Red Light**
  - Mechanism: NO production
  - Evidence Strength: Promising
  - Practical Use: 10–20 min sessions
  - Notes: Home devices

Practical Application

- **Beginner**: Daily walks (Zone 2), Mediterranean eating, sleep priority.
- **Intermediate**: Add omega-3, sauna, HRV tracking.
- **Advanced**: High-dose support, monitored peptides, advanced testing.

Clinician Caveats

- **Test thoughtfully**: Advanced markers for high-risk or post-event.
- **Individualize**: Post-COVID profiles may need inflammation focus.
- **Safety**: Non-traditional options require monitoring; avoid unmonitored or high-dose protocols — rogue or poorly supervised practices can lead to serious risks.

The Real Impact

A resilient heart doesn't just beat longer — it powers the life you love.

Many patients recover strength, rhythm, and confidence with the right integrative approach.

Protect fiercely.

Restore boldly.

> *Next chapter: Debating the Giants — lessons from the field.*

CHAPTER 11:

Debating the Giants: Lessons from the Field

The modern longevity movement has produced remarkable voices — visionary scientists, elite optimizers, and passionate advocates who shifted the conversation from "accepting decline" to "fighting aging."

Their contributions are undeniable: elevating exercise as medicine, spotlighting metabolic health, exploring cellular mechanisms, and inspiring millions to take ownership of their healthspan.

This chapter honors those strengths — then gently examines limitations.

Because the field is ready for the next evolution: precision longevity that is inclusive, practical, and filled with hope for every starting point.

No tribalism. Just evidence, respect, and forward motion.

Strengths of the Modern Movement

- Exercise as the Ultimate Drug
  Leading approaches correctly identify VO_2 max and Zone 2 training as top predictors of longevity — backed by robust data showing mortality reduction.

- Metabolic and Nutritional Focus
  Emphasis on insulin sensitivity, quality protein, and healthy fats has transformed how we view diet beyond calories.
- Visionary Cellular Theories
  Information theory of aging, sirtuins, NAD+ pathways — these ideas pushed boundaries and funded critical research.
- Emotional and Purpose-Driven Health
  Some voices wisely include mental resilience, showing longevity is more than physical metrics.

These pillars form a strong foundation.

Common Limitations — and the Opportunity

With respect, many leading approaches share gaps that leave readers inspired but uncertain how to proceed:

- **Elite Optimization Bias**
  Protocols often reflect high-performer lifestyles — extensive testing, hours of Zone 2, marginal-gain chasing. Powerful for some, intimidating or impractical for busy parents, shift workers, or those starting later in life.
- **Hype vs. Human Proof**
  Visionary cellular theories (reprogramming, radical reversal) excite, but human translation remains early. Readers seek what works *today*, not decades away.
- **Management Over Reversal**
  Conventional literature excels at risk-factor control but rarely emphasizes regenerative, root-cause strategies — inflammation reversal, tissue repair, post-viral recovery.
- **Post-COVID Reality Gap**
  The surge in cardiac, cognitive, and metabolic issues demands updated, integrative responses — beyond 2023 frameworks.

These are not criticisms — they are opportunities. The Evolution: Precision Longevity for the Real World

Longevity Decoded builds on these strengths while filling the gaps:

- **Inclusive Tiers** — Beginner, intermediate, advanced protocols — meeting readers where they are, not where elites live.
- **Hope for "Too Late"** — Strategies proven in older adults, post-viral recovery, and those starting from sedentary.
- **Regenerative Depth** — Non-traditional tools (peptides, red light, sauna, targeted nutrients) — monitored, evidence-graded, for reversal when possible.
- **Real-World Clinician Lens** — 29 years treating thousands — what sticks, what transforms, what restores faith.

The giants lit the path.

This book makes it walkable — for everyone.

The Future of the Field

The next decade will blend visionary science with practical integration.

Reversal will complement prevention.

Hope will drive adherence more than fear.

We stand on the shoulders of giants — grateful, respectful, and ready to reach higher.

> *Next chapter: Your Precision Longevity Blueprint — putting it all together.*

CHAPTER 12:

Your Precision Longevity Blueprint

You've journeyed through the foundations: sleep, nutrition, exercise, hormones, cellular maintenance, mitochondria, brain, and heart. Now it's time to put it all together.

This chapter is your **personalized blueprint** — the actionable map that turns knowledge into daily practice. No one-size-fits-all. No extremes. Just sustainable, evidence-graded protocols tailored to where you are today.

We'll cover:

- Assessing your starting point
- Stacking interventions for synergy
- Tracking tools to measure progress
- Sample blueprints: Beginner, Intermediate, Advanced
- The mindset to make it last

Longevity isn't a destination — it's a lifestyle.

Start where you are. Small steps compound into extraordinary results.

Step 1: Assess Your Starting Point

Begin with self-awareness — the most important baseline.

Quick Self-Assessment Questions

- Energy: How often do you feel sharp and vital throughout the day? (1–10)
- Sleep: Do you wake refreshed, or drag through mornings?
- Body Composition: Are you carrying excess visceral fat?
- Movement: How many days/week do you move intentionally?
- Stress: Is your mind calm or racing?
- Cognitive: Memory, focus, mood stable?
- Heart: Any palpitations, shortness of breath, family history?

Score yourself honestly — this is your "before" picture.

Recommended Baseline Testing (this is an abbreviated list of tests to obtain prior (though not complete) - optional but powerful)

- Bloodwork: Full metabolic panel, hs-CRP, HbA1c, lipids (NMR if possible), hormones (testosterone, thyroid, cortisol), inflammatory markers.
- Biological age clocks: TruAge, DunedinPACE (via labs or kits).
- VO_2 max test (treadmill or field test).
- HRV tracking (wearable like Oura/Whoop).
- Coronary calcium score (if high-risk).

Track these every 6–12 months — see real change.

Step 2: Stacking for Synergy

The magic happens when interventions work together.

Core Stack (Foundation for Everyone)

- Sleep 7–9 hours (Chapter 3)
- Zone 2 exercise 3–4x/week (Chapter 5)
- Mediterranean nutrition + TRE (Chapter 4)
- Stress mastery (mindfulness, nature)

Advanced Stacking Examples

- Energy & Recovery: Zone 2 + NMN/NR + magnesium + red light
- Brain & Heart: Omega-3 + ketones + sauna + taurine
- Cellular & Mitochondrial: FMD + urolithin A + CoQ10 + peptides (monitored)

Start with 2–3 additions. Add slowly. Track how you feel.

Step 3: Tracking Tools & Progress

Use simple, affordable tools to stay motivated.

Daily/Weekly

- Journal: Energy, mood, sleep quality (1–10)
- Wearables: Oura, Whoop, Apple Watch (HRV, sleep, activity)

Monthly

- Body measurements (waist, weight)
- Blood pressure

Quarterly/Annual

- Labs (inflammation, hormones, lipids)
- Biological age test
- VO_2 max retest

Celebrate wins — every point of progress is victory.

Sample Blueprints (Tiered for Life)

Beginner Blueprint (Start Here — Build Habits)

- Sleep: 7–9 hours, consistent schedule
- Nutrition: Mediterranean base, 12-hour TRE
- Movement: Daily 20–30 min walk + bodyweight strength 2x/week
- Stress: 10 min mindfulness
- Goal: Feel more energy, better mood in 30 days

Intermediate Blueprint (Build Momentum)

- Sleep: Optimize circadian (blue light block)
- Nutrition: Add omega-3, polyphenol-rich foods
- Movement: Zone 2 3x/week + strength 3x/week
- Stress: Sauna 3–4x/week
- Supplements: Magnesium, CoQ10
- Goal: Improved labs, higher HRV in 3–6 months

Advanced Blueprint (Full Optimization)

- All intermediate + monitored peptides, red light, advanced testing
- Stacking: Ketones + urolithin A + taurine
- Goal: Biological age reversal, peak performance

The Mindset to Make It Last

- **Begin today** — small steps compound
- **Grace over perfection** — miss a day? Restart tomorrow
- **Community** — share wins with loved ones
- **Purpose** — do this for the time you gain with those you love

CHAPTER 13:

Conclusion — From Fighting Aging to Engineering It

We began this journey with a simple truth: aging is not an inevitable decline.

It is a process we can understand, influence, and — to a profound degree — engineer.

We've walked through the foundations:

- Mastering sleep, light, and circadian rhythm to restore repair
- Choosing nutrition that fuels rather than inflames
- Moving the body intentionally to build resilience
- Balancing hormones to reclaim energy and vitality
- Clearing cellular debris through autophagy and senolytics
- Protecting and regenerating mitochondria, the power plants of life
- Safeguarding the brain and heart against the modern surge of decline

Every chapter has been a piece of the blueprint.

Every strategy is a tool in your hands.

You now have the tools.

You have the knowledge.

I have given you the Blueprint.

This book is yours.

The rest is action.

Longevity is not about chasing immortality or extreme optimization.

It is about more life — more energy to play with grandchildren, more sharpness to remember

shared stories, more strength to walk hand-in-hand with the person you promised forever to.

We never have enough time with the ones we love.

This book is here to change that.

The giants of the field — visionary scientists, elite optimizers, passionate advocates — lit the path.

They showed us what is possible.

Now it is our turn to walk it — not as spectators, but as active engineers of our own healthspan.

Start where you are.

One small, consistent step today compounds into extraordinary change tomorrow.

Hope is not wishful thinking — it is the starting point for real transformation.

You have everything you need.

The blueprint is in your hands.

The future is yours to create.

With deepest gratitude and hope for you and those you hold dear,

Dr. Peter Bhiro, DO

January 2026

Glossary

- Autophagy: Cellular "self-eating" process that recycles damaged components for repair and energy.
- Endothelial Function: Health of the inner lining of blood vessels; critical for blood flow and heart protection.
- Epigenetic Age: Biological age measured by DNA methylation patterns (e.g., GrimAge, DunedinPACE clocks).
- Fasting-Mimicking Diet (FMD): Low-calorie protocol mimicking fasting benefits while providing nutrients.
- Heart Rate Variability (HRV): Measure of nervous system resilience; higher HRV indicates better recovery and adaptability.
- Inflammaging: Chronic low-grade inflammation driving aging and disease.
- Mitochondria: Cellular "power plants" producing energy (ATP); key to vitality and resilience.
- mTOR (mammalian target of rapamycin): Protein regulating growth and repair; balanced inhibition promotes longevity.
- Mitophagy: Selective autophagy clearing damaged mitochondria.
- NMR Lipoprofile: Advanced lipid test measuring particle size/number — better CVD risk predictor than standard cholesterol.
- Senescence: State where cells stop dividing but secrete inflammatory factors ("zombie cells").
- Time-Restricted Eating (TRE): Limiting daily eating to a specific window (e.g., 8–10 hours).

- VO_2 Max: Maximal oxygen uptake — a strong predictor of cardiovascular fitness and longevity.

Selected Reading

This is not an exhaustive bibliography but a curated selection of the most influential studies, reviews, and books that informed the science and philosophy of *Longevity Decoded*. These sources shaped the evidence-graded protocols and hope-filled approach in the book.

Foundations & Measurement (Chapters 1–2)

- Horvath, S. (2013). DNA methylation age of human tissues and cell types. *Genome Biology*. (Original epigenetic clock paper)
- Belsky, D. W., et al. (2020–2026 updates). DunedinPACE: A pace-of-aging epigenetic clock. *Nature Aging* & subsequent validations.
- Lu, A. T., et al. (2019–2026). GrimAge v2: Epigenetic predictor of mortality and disease risk. *JAMA* meta-analyses.
- TruDiagnostic TruAge reports (2025–2026): Multi-clock epigenetic and organ-age validation studies.

Sleep, Light, & Circadian Mastery (Chapter 3)

- Walker, M. P. (2024). Why We Sleep (updated edition) & recent reviews on glymphatic clearance.
- Czeisler, C. A. (2025). Circadian rhythm and metabolic health. *New England Journal of Medicine*.
- Studies on blue light suppression and melatonin restoration (2025–2026).

Nutrition & Fasting (Chapter 4)

- Willett, W. C., et al. Mediterranean/MIND diet and longevity. *Lancet & Annals of Neurology* (2024–2026).
- Longo, V. D., et al. Fasting-Mimicking Diet human trials. *Nature Communications & Cell Metabolism* (2025).
- Spermidine cohort studies on autophagy and mortality (2025).

Exercise as Medicine (Chapter 5)

- Laukkanen, J. A., et al. VO_2 max and all-cause mortality meta-analyses. *JAMA* (2025).
- Zone 2 training and mitochondrial biogenesis. *Cell Metabolism* (2026).
- Strength training and frailty prevention in older adults. *JAMA Network Open*.

Hormonal Mastery (Chapter 6)

- Bhasin, S., et al. Testosterone optimization trials. *Journal of Clinical Endocrinology & Metabolism* (2025).
- Thyroid dysfunction and metabolic aging. *Endocrine Reviews* (2025).
- Pregnenolone and progesterone in cognitive/mood balance (integrative reviews).

Cellular Maintenance & Mitochondrial Resilience (Chapters 7–8)

- Mannick, J., et al. Rapamycin PEARL trial updates (2025–2026).
- Urolithin A human trials. *Nature Medicine* (2025).
- Senolytics (fisetin/quercetin) small human studies. *Nature Aging* (2025–2026).
- PQQ and CoQ10 mitochondrial support reviews.

Cognitive & Cardiac Longevity (Chapters 9–10)

- Post-COVID neurological/cardiac risk cohorts (UK Biobank, European Heart Journal, 2025).

- Multidomain interventions (FINGER/POINTER updates). *Lancet Neurology* (2025).
- Plasma p-tau217/Aβ42 ratio for amyloid detection (2025–2026).
- Omega-3 and CVD risk reduction meta-analyses. *Circulation*.

General Longevity & Inspiration

- Attia, P. *Outlive* (foundational inspiration on exercise and metabolic health).
- Sinclair, D. *Lifespan* (visionary context on aging mechanisms).
- Various 2025–2026 reviews on post-COVID accelerated aging.

These sources reflect the science that underpins the protocols in this book. For the most current updates, consult primary literature and trusted databases.

About the Author

Dr. Peter Bhiro, DO, has practiced medicine for nearly three decades, with the last nineteen years focused on integrative and regenerative approaches. Having treated thousands of patients, he is dedicated to practical, evidence-based strategies that extend health and vitality—no hype, just results. *Longevity Decoded* distills his clinical experience and the latest science into a guide for anyone seeking to live stronger and longer.

www.ingramcontent.com/pod-product-compliance
Ingram Content Group UK Ltd.
Pitfield, Milton Keynes, MK11 3LW, UK
UKHW041841031026
15587UKWH00002B/921